TYPE 1 DIABETES COOKBOOK FOR BEGINNERS

Delicious & Healthy Recipes for Type 1 Diabetics

By

Jade Hanson

Table of Contents

INTRODUCTION

Type 1 diabetes is a chronic condition that requires careful management and monitoring of blood sugar levels. One of the most important ways to manage type 1 diabetes is through proper nutrition and meal planning. Eating a healthy and balanced diet not only helps regulate blood sugar levels but also provides the necessary nutrients for overall health and wellness.

However, meal planning for type 1 diabetes can be overwhelming, especially for those just starting out on their journey. That's why we created this cookbook - to make meal planning and eating for type 1 diabetes easier and more accessible for everyone.

In this cookbook, you'll find delicious and easy-to-prepare recipes, along with tips for meal planning and blood sugar management. We'll cover everything from understanding carbohydrates and blood sugar management, to planning healthy meals and incorporating treats and desserts into your diet.

Whether you're a beginner or just looking for new ideas, this cookbook is the perfect resource for anyone looking to take control of their type 1 diabetes through a healthy and balanced diet. So, let's get started on your journey towards better health and wellness today!

CHAPTER ONE

Understanding Carbohydrates and Blood Sugar Management

Type 1 diabetes requires careful management of blood sugar levels, and this is largely achieved through monitoring and controlling carbohydrate intake. This chapter will provide an in-depth look at carbohydrates, their impact on blood sugar levels, and strategies for managing blood sugar through carb counting and meal planning.

How Carbs Affect Blood Sugar

Carbohydrates are the primary source of energy in our diet, and they are broken down into glucose (sugar) in the body. When we eat carbohydrates, the glucose is released into the bloodstream, causing blood sugar levels to rise. For individuals with type 1 diabetes, this process can be challenging as the body does not produce insulin to regulate the glucose levels. Instead, individuals with type 1 diabetes must carefully monitor their carbohydrate intake and use insulin injections to keep their blood sugar levels in check.

Understanding Carb Counting

Carb counting is a way of tracking the number of carbohydrates you consume in each meal. By knowing the number of carbs you consume, you can better control your blood sugar levels and avoid highs and lows. To get started with carb counting, you'll need to learn how many grams of carbohydrates are in the foods you eat. This information can be found on food labels, online databases, and in carbohydrate counting books.

Strategies for Managing Blood Sugar

In addition to carb counting, there are several other strategies you can use to help manage blood sugar levels. For example:

- Eating regular meals and snacks at the same time each day
- Staying active throughout the day
- Monitoring blood sugar levels regularly
- Adjusting insulin doses based on blood sugar levels and food intake
- Seeking guidance from a healthcare provider

Working with a Healthcare Provider

Managing type 1 diabetes can be challenging, but having the right support and resources can make a big difference. Working with a healthcare provider can help you create a personalized plan for managing your blood sugar levels and eating a healthy diet. Your healthcare provider can also provide guidance on insulin dosing, monitoring blood sugar levels, and managing any complications that may arise.

CHAPTER TWO

Meal Planning 101

Meal planning is an important aspect of managing type 1 diabetes. Proper meal planning helps keep blood sugar levels in check and provides the necessary nutrients for overall health. In this chapter, we will cover the basics of meal planning and offer tips for making meal planning a part of your daily routine.

How to Plan Healthy Meals:

Create a weekly grocery list to get started. Plan for three main meals (breakfast, lunch, and dinner) and snacks.

Make sure to include a variety of foods from all food groups, including whole grains, lean proteins, healthy fats, and fresh fruits and vegetables.

Try to incorporate at least two or three servings of non-starchy vegetables into each meal.

Choose lean protein sources, such as chicken, turkey, fish, and legumes.

Use healthy oils, such as olive oil or avocado oil, when cooking or preparing meals.

Tips for Meal Prep and Batch Cooking:

Cook once, eat twice. Cook larger portions of meals and save leftovers for later in the week.

Invest in containers for food storage. This makes it easy to pack meals for work or school.

Prepare healthy snacks, such as cut up fruits and veggies, in advance.

Use a slow cooker to prepare meals, such as soups and stews, for easy and convenient meals during the week.

Ideas for Quick and Easy Meals:

Turkey or chicken salad with whole grain crackers
Veggie and hummus wrap
Grilled chicken or fish with roasted vegetables
Greek yogurt topped with berries and honey
Baked sweet potato with almond butter and a side of steamed broccoli

How to Incorporate Treats and Desserts into Your Meal Plan:

Limit treats and desserts to one serving per day.
Choose lower-carb options, such as sorbet or dark chocolate, as a sweet treat.
Use portion control when eating treats and desserts.

Meal planning takes time and effort, but the benefits of a well-planned diet are worth it. With these tips and ideas, meal planning for type 1 diabetes can be manageable and enjoyable. By incorporating a variety of healthy foods and managing portion sizes, you can keep your blood sugar levels in check and maintain a healthy and balanced diet.

CHAPTER THREE

Breakfast Recipes

1.Oatmeal with Berries and Nuts

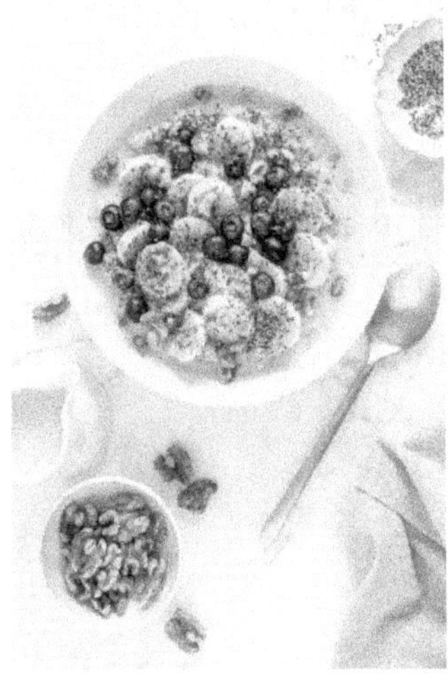

Ingredients:

1 cup of rolled oats

1 cup of unsweetened almond milk

a half-cup of berries (fresh or frozen)

1 tablespoon of chopped nuts (almonds, walnuts, pecans, etc.)

1 teaspoon of pure maple syrup (optional)

Instructions:

- In a saucepan, bring the almond milk to a boil.
- Stir in the oats after lowering the heat to medium-low.
- Cook, stirring occasionally, for about 5 minutes or until the oats are soft and creamy.
- Add in the mixed berries and cook for another minute.
- Remove from heat and stir in the chopped nuts and maple syrup (if using).
- Serve in a bowl and enjoy!

2. Veggie and Cheese Frittata

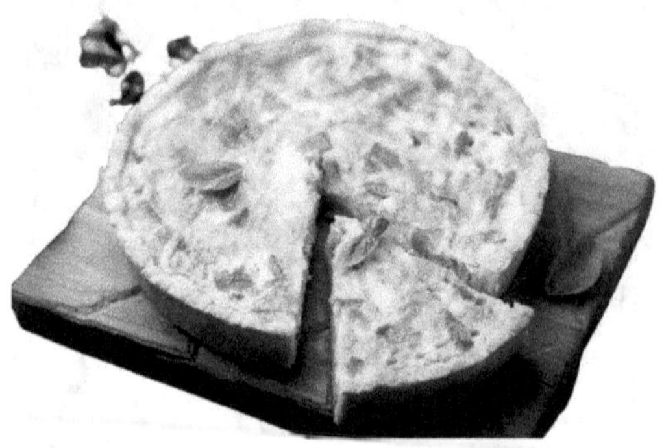

Ingredients:

4 large eggs
1/2 cup of chopped vegetables (bell peppers, onions, mushrooms, etc.)
1/4 cup of grated cheese (cheddar, feta, goat, etc.)
Salt and pepper to taste

1 teaspoon of olive oil.

Instructions:

- Preheat the oven to 375°F.
- The olive oil should be heated over medium heat in a sizable oven-safe skillet.
- Add the chopped vegetables and cook until they are soft and tender, about 5 minutes.
- Salt and pepper the eggs and whisk them in a sizable mixing dish.
- The eggs should be poured over the skillet's vegetables.
- Grate the cheese over the top of the eggs.
- Place the skillet in the oven and bake for about 15 minutes or until the eggs are set and the cheese is melted.
- Slice into wedges and serve hot

3. Greek Yogurt Parfait

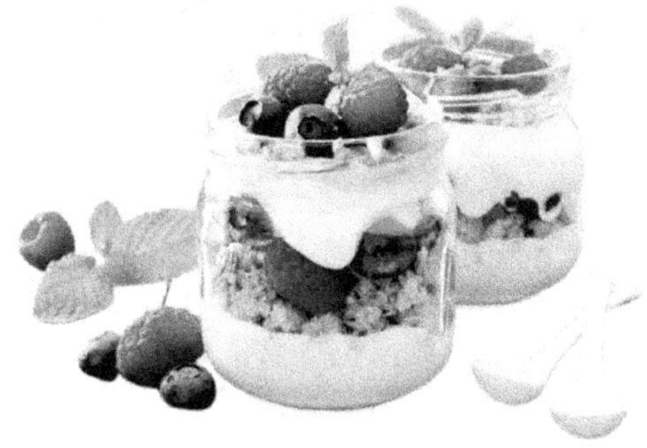

Ingredients:

1 cup of Greek yogurt
a half-cup of berries (fresh or frozen)
1/4 cup of granola
1 tablespoon of honey (optional)

Instructions:

- In a glass or bowl, layer the Greek yogurt, mixed berries, and granola.
- Drizzle with honey (if using) and enjoy!

4. Whole Grain Pancakes with Fresh Berries

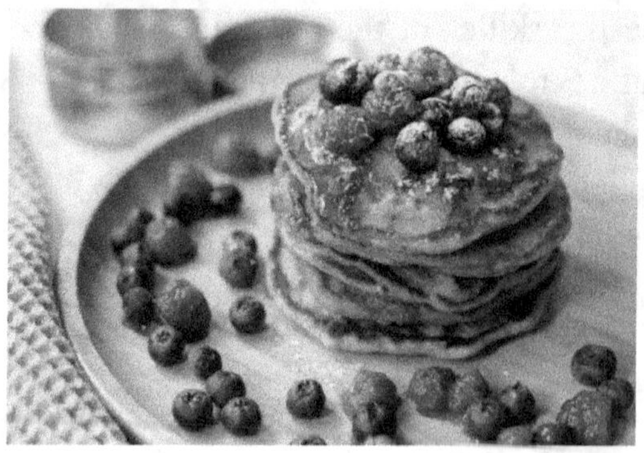

Ingredients:

1 cup of whole wheat flour
1 teaspoon of baking powder
1/2 teaspoon of baking soda
1/4 teaspoon of salt
1 large egg

1 cup of unsweetened almond milk

1 tablespoon of pure maple syrup

a half-cup of berries (fresh or frozen)

Instructions:

- Mix the flour, baking soda, salt, and baking powder in a big bowl.
- In another bowl, beat the egg, almond milk, and maple syrup.
- After adding the liquid components, mix the dry ingredients only until they are barely blended.
- Heat a non-stick pan over medium heat.
- Using a 1/4 cup measure, pour the batter into the pan and sprinkle with a few berries.
- Cook for about 2-3 minutes on each side or until golden brown.
- Repeat with the remaining batter and serve with additional fresh berries.

5. Avocado Toast with Fried Egg

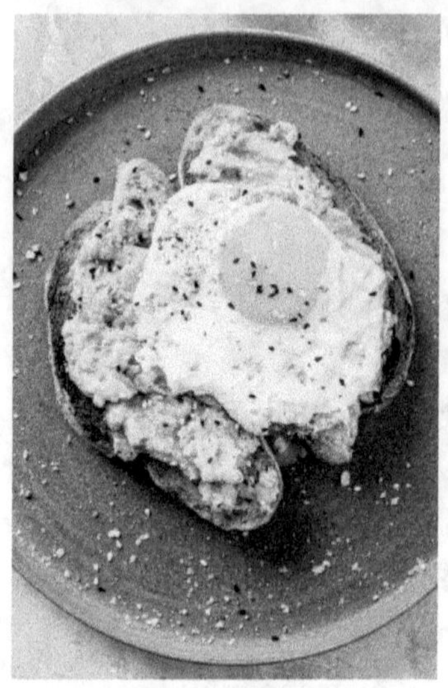

Ingredients:

2 slices of whole grain bread.
1 ripe avocado.
Salt and pepper to taste.
2 large eggs.
1 teaspoon of olive oil.

Instructions:

- Toast the bread to your liking.
- Remove the avocado pit by cutting into half
- Mash the avocado and spread it over the toasted bread.
- Season with salt and pepper to taste.

- A small skillet should be placed over medium heat to warm the olive oil.
- Crack the eggs into the skillet and cook until the whites are set but the yolks are still runny, about 2-3 minutes.
- Place one fried egg on top of each slice of avocado toast and serve immediately.

6. Peanut Butter Banana Smoothie

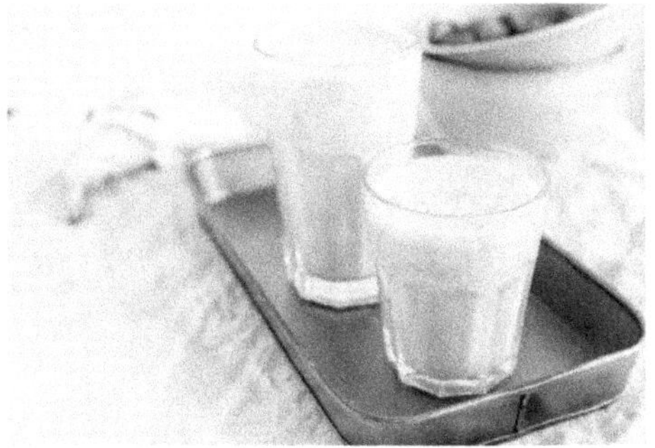

Ingredients:

1 ripe banana
1/2 cup of unsweetened almond milk
1/4 cup of Greek yogurt
1 tablespoon of natural peanut butter
1 scoop of protein powder (optional)
1/2 teaspoon of vanilla extract.

Instructions:

- In a blender, combine the banana, almond milk, Greek yogurt, peanut butter, protein powder (if using), and vanilla extract.
- Blend till smooth and creamy at high speed.
- Pour into a glass and enjoy!

7. Tofu Scramble with Vegetables

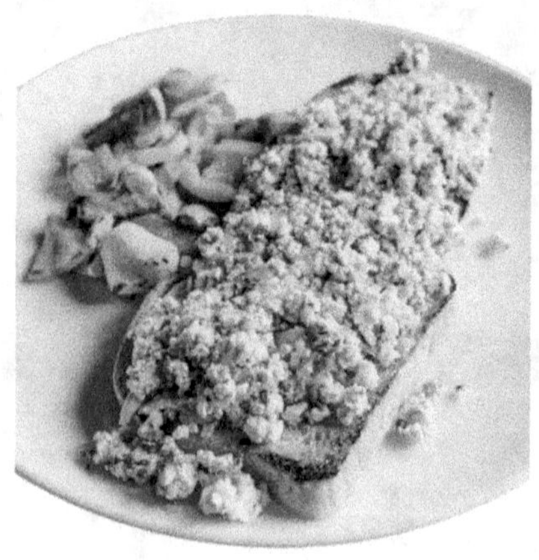

Ingredients:

1 block of firm tofu
1/2 cup of chopped vegetables (bell peppers, onions, mushrooms, etc.)
Salt and pepper to taste
1 teaspoon of olive oil.

Instructions:

- Set aside the tofu crumbles in a bowl.
- A small skillet should be placed over medium heat to warm the olive oil.
- Add the chopped vegetables and cook until they are soft and tender, about 5 minutes.
- Stir in the tofu crumbles after adding it to the skillet.
- Season with salt and pepper to taste.
- Cook for a further 5 minutes, or until well heated.
- Serve hot and enjoy!

8. Whole Grain English Muffin with Egg and Cheese

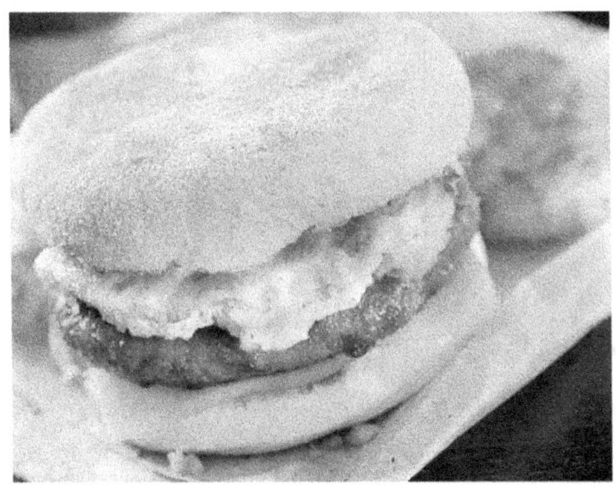

Ingredients:

2 whole grain English muffins
2 large eggs

2 slices of cheese (cheddar, American, etc.)
Salt and pepper to taste
1 teaspoon of butter.

Instructions:

- Toast the English muffins to your liking.
- A small skillet should be placed over medium heat to warm the butter.
- Crack the eggs into the skillet and cook until the whites are set but the yolks are still runny, about 2-3 minutes.
- Place one slice of cheese on top of each English muffin.
- Place one fried egg on top of the cheese on each muffin.
- Season with salt and pepper to taste.
- Serve hot and enjoy!

CHAPTER FOUR

Lunch Recipes

1.Grilled Chicken Salad with Mixed Greens

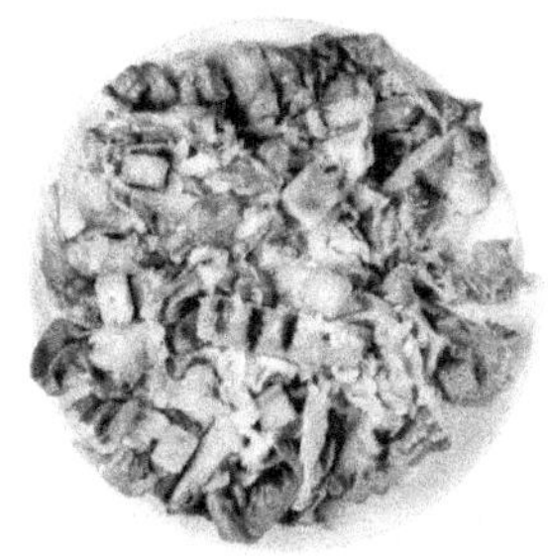

Ingredients:

2 boneless, skinless chicken breasts

Salt and pepper to taste

2 tablespoons of olive oil

4 cups of mixed greens

1/2 cup of cherry tomatoes, halved

1/4 cup of crumbled feta cheese

1/4 cup of balsamic vinaigrette

Instructions:

- Chicken breasts should be salted and peppered.

- In a large skillet set over medium heat, the olive oil needs to warm up.

- Add the chicken breasts to the skillet and cook until they are golden brown on both sides and cooked through, about 4-5 minutes per side.

- The chicken should be taken out of the skillet and given five minutes to rest.

- In a large bowl, combine the mixed greens, cherry tomatoes, and crumbled feta cheese.

- Slice the chicken into strips and add it to the bowl with the greens.

- Toss everything together with the balsamic vinaigrette.

- Serve immediately and enjoy!

2. Turkey and Cheese Wrap with Avocado

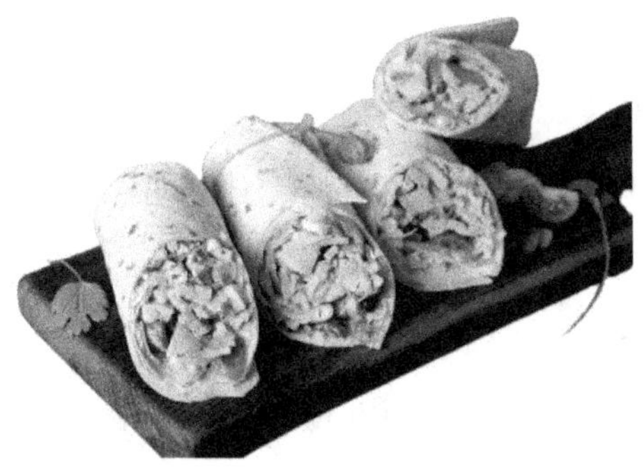

Ingredients:

2 whole grain wraps

4 slices of turkey breast

2 slices of cheese (cheddar, American, etc.)

1 ripe avocado

Salt and pepper to taste

1 tablespoon of mayonnaise.

Instructions:

- Place one wrap on a plate.

- Arrange 2 slices of turkey on the wrap.

- Cut the avocado into half to remove the pit.

- Mash the avocado and spread it over the turkey.

- Sprinkle salt and pepper to taste over the avocado

- Place one slice of cheese on top of the avocado.

- Roll the wrap tightly to form a cylinder.

- Repeat the process with the second wrap.

- Serve each wrap right away after being cut in half.

3. Veggie and Hummus Sandwich

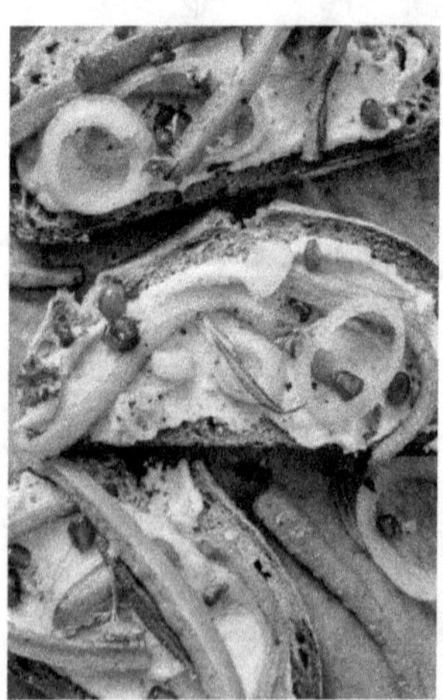

Ingredients:

2 whole grain slices of bread

1/4 cup of hummus

1/2 cup of sliced vegetables (bell peppers, cucumbers, carrots, etc.)

Salt and pepper to taste.

Instructions:

- As desired, toast the bread slices.
- The hummus should be spread on one slice of bread.
- Arrange the sliced vegetables on top of the hummus.
- Salt and pepper should be added to taste to the vegetables.
- To assemble a sandwich, put the second slice of bread on top.
- Serve immediately and enjoy!

4.Quinoa and Black Bean Salad

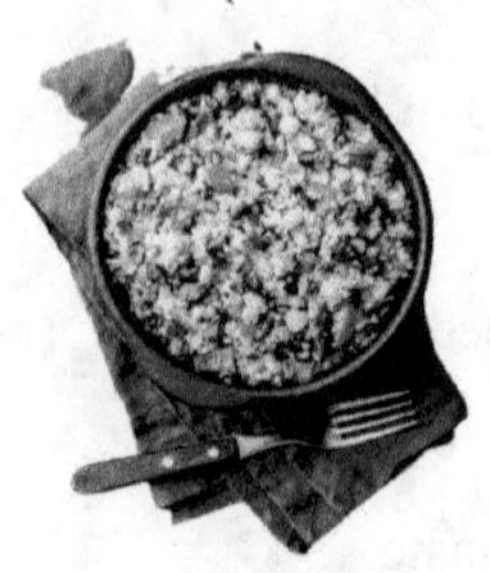

Ingredients:

1 cup of cooked quinoa

one washed and drained can of black beans.

1/2 cup of cherry tomatoes, halved

1/4 cup of red onion, diced

1/4 cup of cilantro, chopped

1 lime, juiced

Salt and pepper to taste

2 tablespoons of olive oil.

Instructions:

- The cooked quinoa, black beans, cherry tomatoes, red onion, and cilantro should all be combined in a big bowl.

- In a small bowl, whisk together the lime juice, salt, pepper, and olive oil to make a dressing.
- Then add the dressing and toss to coat the quinoa and bean combination.
- Serve immediately and enjoy!

5.Tuna Salad Lettuce Wraps

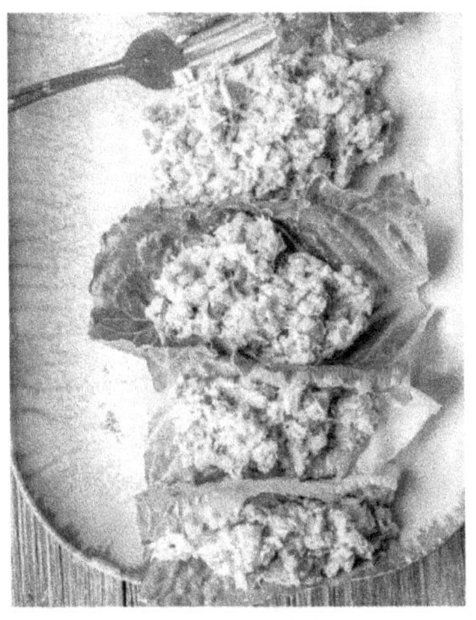

Ingredients:

2 cans of tuna, drained

1/4 cup of mayonnaise

1/4 cup of diced celery

1/4 cup of diced red onion

1/4 cup of diced pickles

Salt and pepper to taste

8 leaves of lettuce (iceberg, romaine, etc.)

Instructions:

- In a large bowl, combine the tuna, mayonnaise, celery, red onion, and pickles.
- To taste, add salt and pepper to the mixture.
- Spoon 2-3 tablespoons of the tuna salad onto each lettuce leaf.
- Roll up the lettuce leaves and serve immediately.

6.Egg Salad Sandwiches

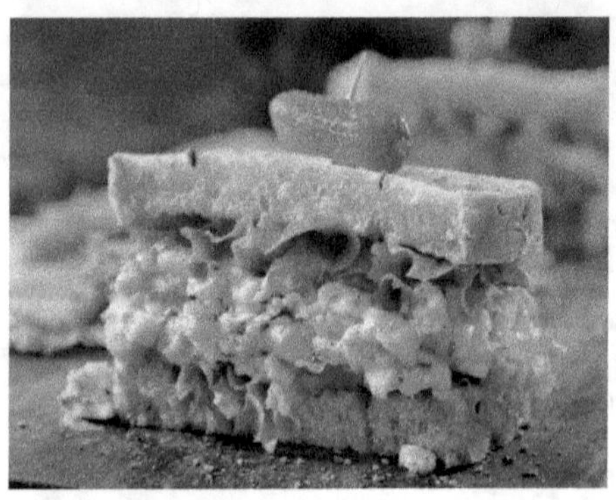

Ingredients:

6 eggs, hard-boiled

1/4 cup of mayonnaise

1 tablespoon of yellow mustard

1/4 cup of diced celery

Salt and pepper to taste

6 slices of whole grain bread.

Instructions:

- Peel and chop the hard-boiled eggs.
- In a large bowl, combine the eggs, mayonnaise, mustard, celery, salt, and pepper.
- Mix everything together until well combined.
- As desired, toast the bread slices.
- Spread the egg salad evenly over three of the slices of bread.
- Top each slice with another slice of bread to make a sandwich.
- Serve immediately and enjoy!

7.Greek Yogurt Chicken Salad

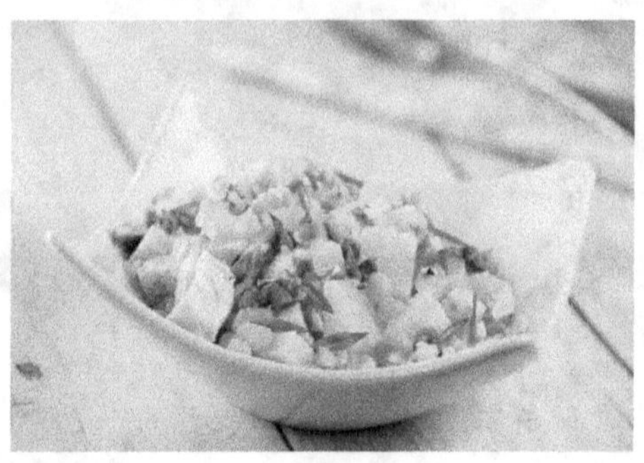

Ingredients:

2 boneless, skinless chicken breasts

Salt and pepper to taste

2 tablespoons of olive oil

1 cup of Greek yogurt

1/4 cup of diced red onion

1/4 cup of diced cucumber

1/4 cup of diced cherry tomatoes

1 tablespoon of lemon juice

8 leaves of lettuce (iceberg, romaine, etc.)

Instructions:

- Chicken breasts should be salted and peppered.

- In a large skillet set over medium heat, the olive oil needs to warm up.

- Add the chicken breasts to the skillet and cook until they are golden brown on both sides and cooked through, about 4-5 minutes per side.

- The chicken should be taken out of the skillet and given five minutes to rest.

- In a large bowl, combine the Greek yogurt, red onion, cucumber, cherry tomatoes, lemon juice, and salt and pepper to taste.

- Cut the chicken into bite-sized pieces and add it to the bowl with the yogurt mixture.

- Toss everything together until well combined.

- Spoon the chicken salad onto the lettuce leaves and serve immediately.

CHAPTER FIVE

Dinner Recipes

1.Baked Salmon with Roasted Veggies

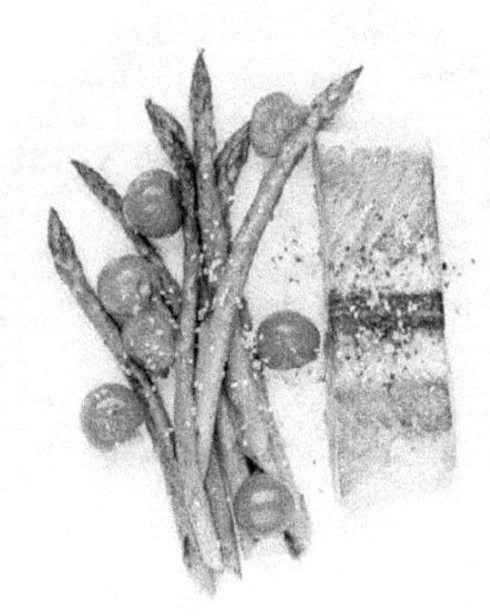

Ingredients:

4 salmon fillets
2 cups of chopped vegetables (e.g., carrots, bell peppers, zucchini)
2 tablespoons of olive oil
Salt and pepper, to taste
Fresh herbs (optional)

Instructions:

- Preheat the oven to 400°F (200°C).
- Line a baking sheet with parchment paper.
- In a large bowl, combine the chopped vegetables with olive oil, salt, pepper, and herbs (if using).
- Arrange the vegetables on one half of the prepared baking sheet.
- Place the salmon fillets on the other half of the baking sheet.
- Bake the salmon for 12 to 15 minutes, or until it is done and the vegetables are soft.

2. Turkey Chili

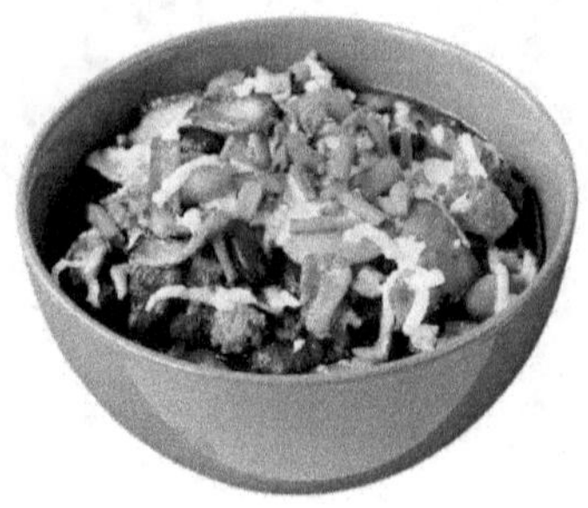

Ingredients:

1 pound of ground turkey

1 large onion, chopped

1 red bell pepper, chopped

3 cloves of garlic, minced

1 can of diced tomatoes (14.5 ounces)

1 can of kidney beans (14.5 ounces), drained and rinsed
1 can of corn (14.5 ounces), drained
2 tablespoons of chili powder
1 teaspoon of cumin
Salt and pepper, to taste

Instructions:

- In a large saucepan, cook the ground turkey over medium heat until browned, about 5-7 minutes.
- Add the chopped onion, red bell pepper, and minced garlic to the pan. Cook the vegetables for 5-7 minutes, or until they are fork-tender.
- Stir in the diced tomatoes, kidney beans, corn, chili powder, cumin, salt, and pepper.
- Bring the chili to a boil, then reduce the heat to low and simmer for 20-30 minutes, stirring occasionally.

3.Spaghetti Squash with Meat Sauce

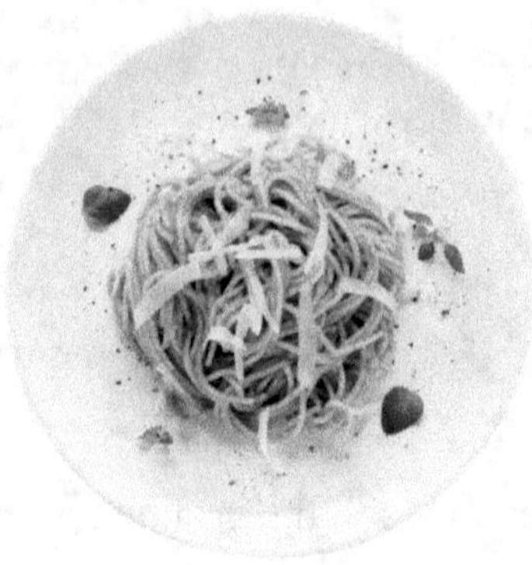

Ingredients:

1 spaghetti squash
1 pound of ground beef
1 large onion, chopped
3 cloves of garlic, minced
1 can of diced tomatoes (14.5 ounces)
1 tablespoon of dried basil
Salt and pepper, to taste

Instructions:

- Preheat the oven to 400°F (200°C).
- Remove the seeds after cutting the spaghetti squash in half lengthwise.
- Squash halves should be placed cut side down on a baking pan.

- The squash should be baked for 30-35 minutes, or until it is tender.
- In a large saucepan, cook the ground beef over medium heat until browned, about 5-7 minutes.
- Add the chopped onion, red bell pepper, and minced garlic to the pan. Cook the vegetables for 5-7 minutes, or until they are fork-tender.
- Stir in the diced tomatoes, basil, salt, and pepper.
- Bring the sauce to a boil, then reduce the heat to low and simmer for 20-30 minutes, stirring occasionally.
- Scrape the spaghetti-like threads from the squash using a fork. Put the beef sauce on top before serving.

4.Grilled Chicken and Vegetable Skewers

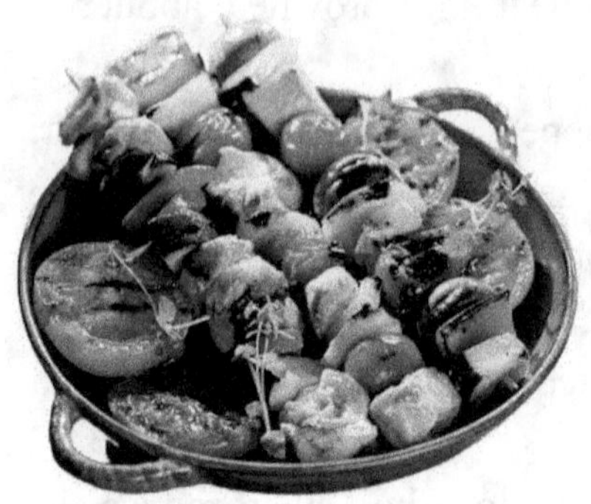

Ingredients:

4 chicken breasts, boneless and skinless, cut into 1-inch cubes.
2 cups of chopped vegetables (e.g., bell peppers, zucchini, onion)
2 tablespoons of olive oil
Salt and pepper, to taste
Fresh herbs (optional)

Instructions:

- 8 wooden skewers should be soaked for at least 30 minutes in water.

- In a large bowl, combine the chicken cubes, chopped vegetables, olive oil, salt, pepper, and herbs (if using).
- Alternately thread the chicken and vegetables onto the skewers.
- Heat a grill pan over medium-high heat.
- Place the skewers on the pan and cook for 8-10 minutes, turning occasionally, until the chicken is cooked through and the vegetables are tender.

5.Baked Potato and Black Bean Enchiladas

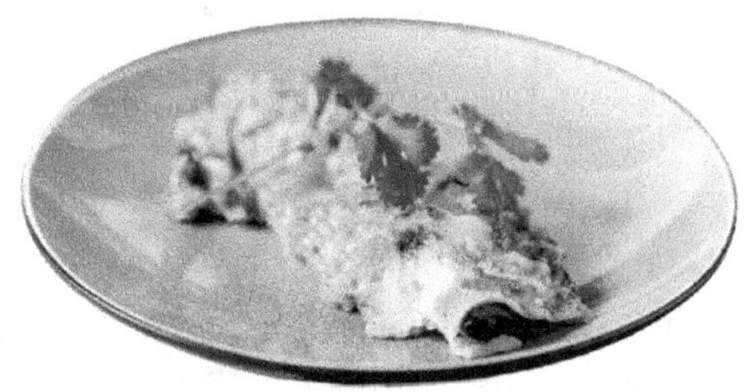

Ingredients:

4 medium russet potatoes, peeled and diced
1 can of rinsed and drained dried black beans.
1 medium onion, diced

2 cloves of garlic, minced
1 cup salsa
1 cup shredded cheddar cheese
8 corn tortillas
Salt and pepper, to taste

Instructions:

- Preheat oven to 375°F (190°C).
- Boil the diced potatoes in a big pot until they are soft. Drain and mash.
- 1 tablespoon of oil should be heated to medium heat in a big skillet. Cooking time for the onion and garlic should be around 5 minutes, or until tender.
- Add the black beans, salsa, and salt and pepper to the skillet and mix well.
- In a 9x13 inch baking dish, spread 1/2 cup of the mashed potatoes in the bottom.
- Lay a tortilla on a flat surface, add a spoonful of the black bean mixture and some of the shredded cheese. Place in the baking dish after rolling up. Repeat with the remaining tortillas.
- Spread the remaining mashed potatoes on top of the enchiladas.
- Bake the dish for 25 minutes with the foil covering.

- Remove the foil and bake for an additional 10 minutes or until the cheese is melted and the edges are slightly crispy.
- Serve hot and enjoy!

6.Grilled Pork Tenderloin with Grilled Vegetables

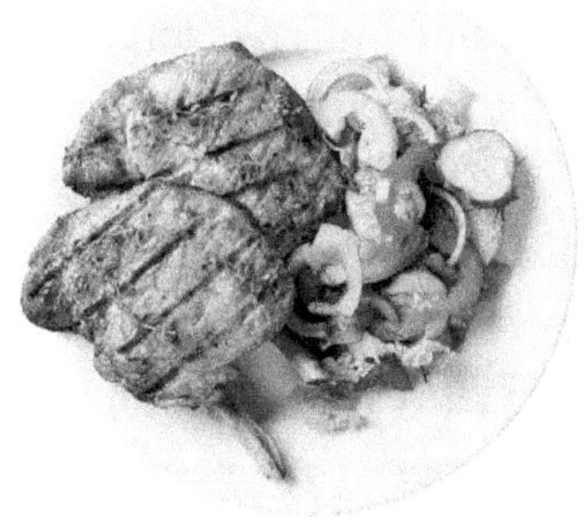

Ingredients:

1 lb. pork tenderloin

1 medium zucchini, sliced

1 medium yellow squash, sliced

1 red bell pepper, sliced

1 yellow bell pepper, sliced

1 red onion, sliced

2 tbsp olive oil

Salt and pepper, to taste.

Instructions:

- Preheat the grill to medium-high heat.
- Brush the pork tenderloin with 1 tbsp of the olive oil and season with salt and pepper.
- In a large bowl, toss the sliced zucchini, yellow squash, red and yellow bell peppers, and red onion with the remaining 1 tbsp of olive oil, salt, and pepper.
- Place the pork on the grill and cook for 10-15 minutes on each side or until the internal temperature reaches 145°F (63°C).
- Place the vegetables on the grill and cook for 10-15 minutes, turning occasionally, until they are slightly charred and tender.
- Remove the pork and vegetables from the grill and let rest for 5 minutes.
- Slice the pork and serve with the grilled vegetables.
- Enjoy!

CHAPTER SIX

Snack Recipes

1.Apple Slices with Peanut Butter:

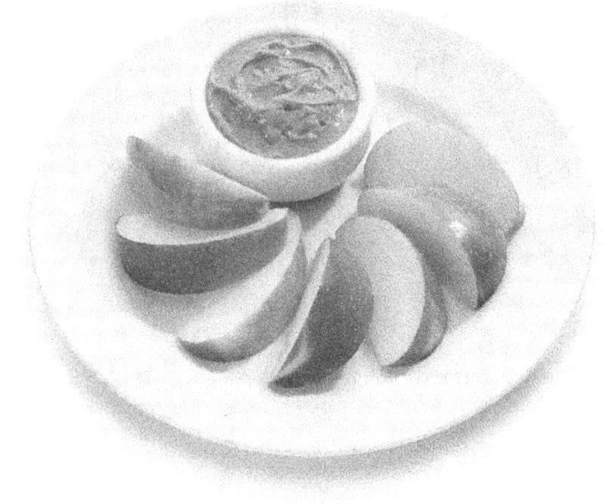

Ingredients:
1 apple, sliced
2 tbsp natural peanut butter

Instructions:
- Arrange the apple slices on a plate.

- Spoon the peanut butter into a small bowl and microwave for 20-30 seconds, or until melted.
- Dip the apple slices into the melted peanut butter for a crunchy and sweet snack.

2.Carrots and Hummus:

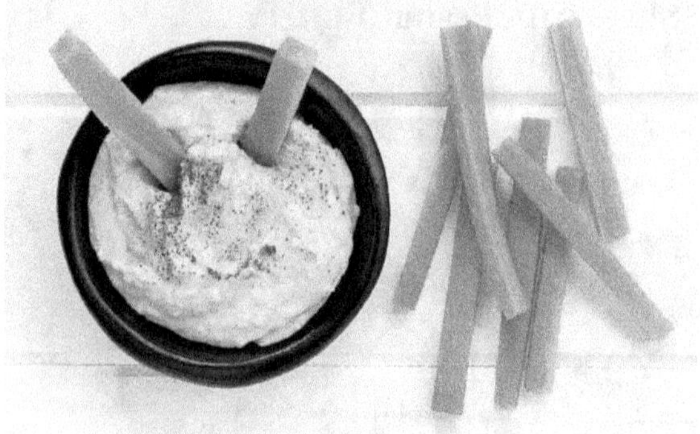

Ingredients:
1 cup hummus
2 carrots, sliced
2 celery sticks, sliced
1 bell pepper, sliced
Instructions:
- Arrange the carrots, celery sticks, and bell pepper on a plate.
- Spoon the hummus into a small bowl.
- Dip the vegetables into the hummus for a crunchy and nutritious snack.

3.Greek Yogurt with Berries:

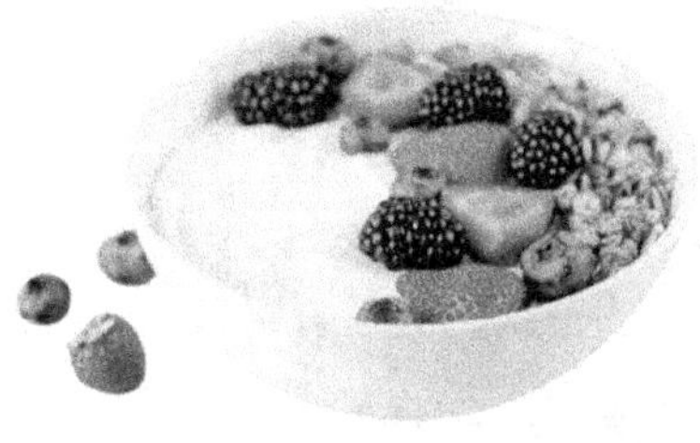

Ingredients:
1 cup Greek yogurt
1/2 cup mixed berries
1/4 cup granola

Instructions:
- Spoon the Greek yogurt into a glass or bowl.
- Top with a layer of mixed berries.
- Sprinkle the granola over the berries.
- Continue adding layers until you reach the glass or bowl's top.
- Serve immediately for a healthy and delicious snack.

4.Roasted Chickpeas:

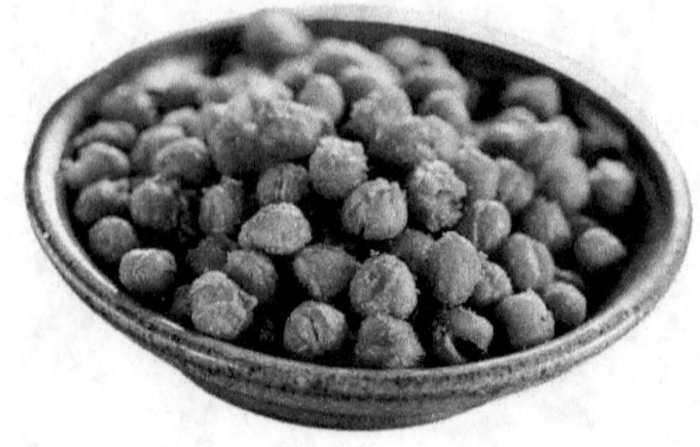

Ingredients:
1 can chickpeas, drained and rinsed
1 tbsp olive oil
Salt, to taste

Instructions:
- Preheat the oven to 400°F (200°C).
- Toss the chickpeas with the olive oil in a big basin.
- Spread the chickpeas out in a single layer on a baking sheet.
- Bake for 20-30 minutes, or until crispy.
- Take out of the oven and season with salt to taste.
- Serve as a snack or sprinkle over a salad for added crunch.

5.Trail Mix:

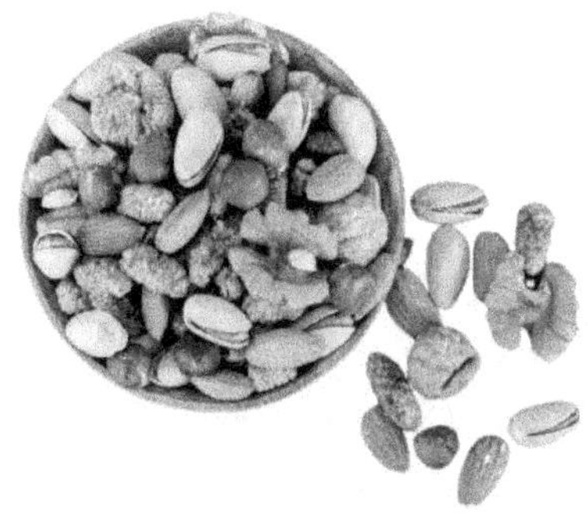

Ingredients:

one cup of mixed nuts (almonds, walnuts, pecans, etc.)

50 g of dried fruit (raisins, cranberries, apricots, etc.)

1/4 cup chocolate chips

Instructions:

- In a large bowl, mix the nuts, dried fruit, and chocolate chips together.
- Serve as a snack or sprinkle over a yogurt parfait for added crunch.

6. Rice Cakes with Banana and Almond Butter:

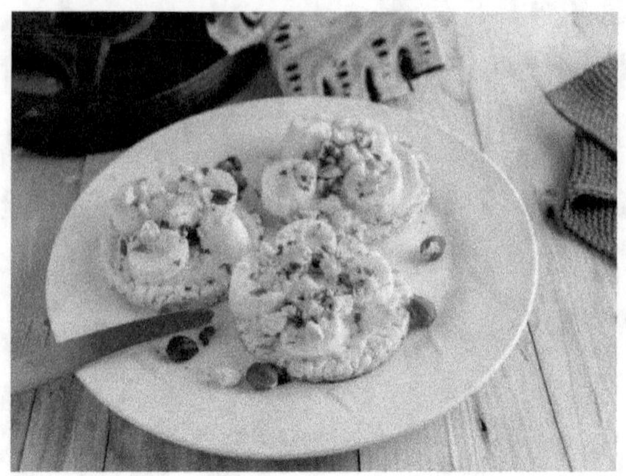

Ingredients:

4 rice cakes

4 tbsp almond butter

2 ripe bananas, sliced

Instructions:

- Toast the rice cakes in a toaster or under a broiler until they are crispy.
- Each rice cake should have 1 tablespoon of almond butter on it.
- On top of the almond butter, arrange the sliced bananas.
- Serve and enjoy as a snack or light meal.

7. Cucumber and Tomato Salad:

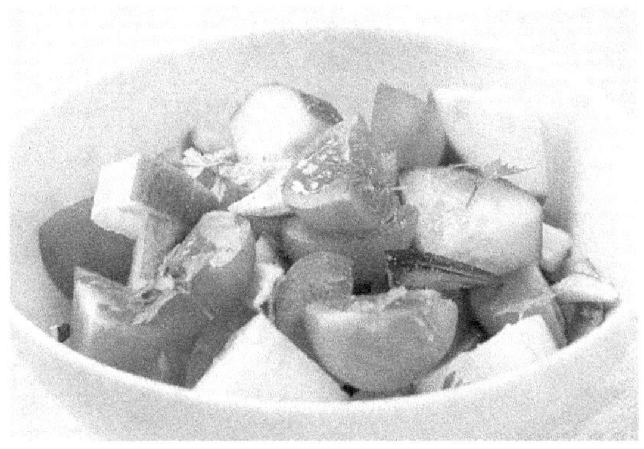

Ingredients:

1 large cucumber, sliced
1 large tomato, diced
2 tbsp balsamic vinegar
Salt, to taste

Instructions:

- In a large bowl, mix the cucumber and tomato together.
- Drizzle with the balsamic vinegar.
- Sprinkle with salt to taste.
- Serve as a snack or as a side dish with a grilled entree.

CHAPTER SEVEN

Dessert Recipes

1.Berry Sorbet

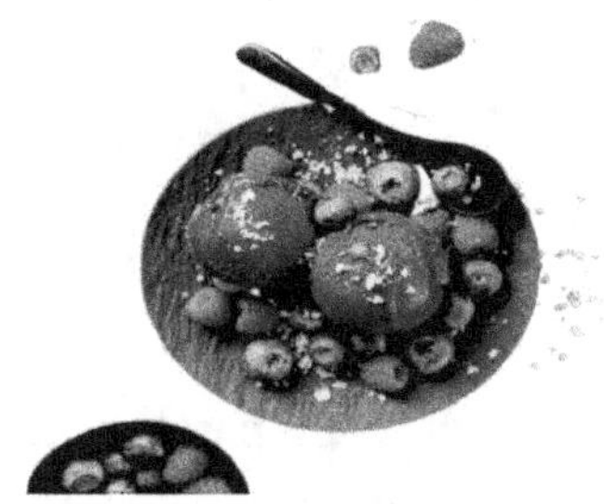

Ingredients: fresh mixed berries, sugar, water, lemon juice

Directions: Blend together mixed berries, sugar, water, and lemon juice until smooth.After putting the mixture in a container, freeze it for several hours. Scoop into bowls and serve.

2. Dark Chocolate Bark with Nuts

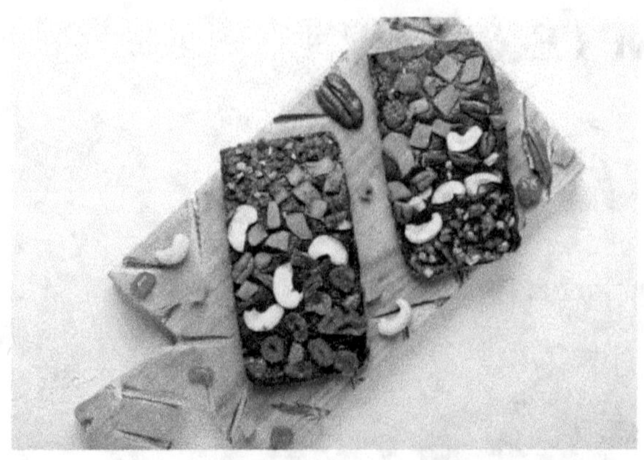

Ingredients: dark chocolate, mixed nuts, sea salt

Directions: Line a baking sheet with parchment paper. Use a double boiler or a microwave to melt the dark chocolate. Pour melted chocolate onto the lined baking sheet and sprinkle with mixed nuts and sea salt. Freezing it for 30 minutes will help it become firm. Break into pieces and serve.

3.Baked Apple Slices

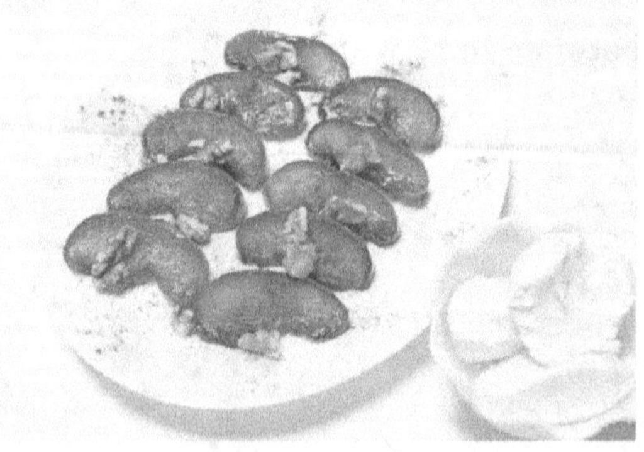

Ingredients: apples, cinnamon, nutmeg, brown sugar, lemon juice

Directions: Preheat oven to 375°F. Slice apples and place them in a single layer on a baking sheet. Sprinkle with cinnamon, nutmeg, brown sugar, and lemon juice. Bake for 15-20 minutes until apples are tender and the edges are slightly caramelized. Serve warm.

4.Flourless Chocolate Brownies

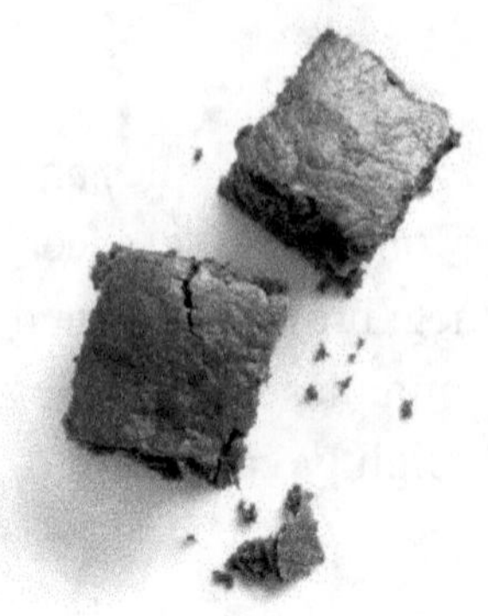

Ingredients: dark chocolate, eggs, sugar, vanilla extract, cocoa powder, salt

Directions: Preheat oven to 350°F. Line a baking dish 8x8 inch with parchment paper. Use a double boiler or a microwave to melt the dark chocolate. In a separate bowl, beat eggs, sugar, and vanilla extract until light and fluffy. Stir in melted chocolate, cocoa powder, and salt until well combined. Pour mixture into the prepared baking dish. Bake for 25-30 minutes until set. Allow to cool completely before slicing.

5.Banana Oat Cookies

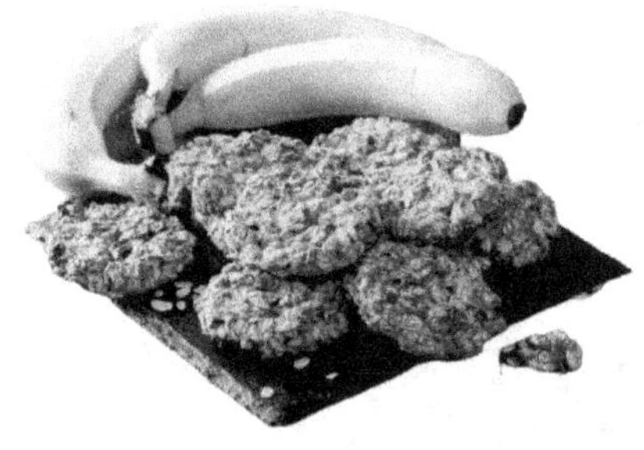

Ingredients: oats, bananas, almond butter, honey, cinnamon, baking powder, baking soda, salt

Directions: Preheat oven to 375°F. In a large bowl, mash bananas and mix in almond butter, honey, cinnamon, baking powder, baking soda, and salt until well combined. Stir in oats until mixture is sticky. Spoonfuls should be dropped onto a parchment-lined baking sheet. Golden brown edges can be achieved by baking for 15-20 minutes. Prior to transferring to a wire rack, give the baked goods five minutes to cool on the baking sheet.

6.Almond Butter Fudge

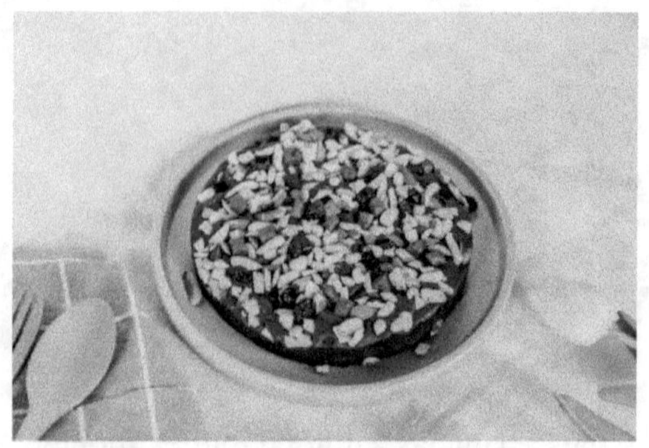

Ingredients: almond butter, coconut oil, honey, vanilla extract, salt

Directions: Line a baking dish 8x8 inch with parchment paper. In a saucepan, melt together almond butter, coconut oil, honey, vanilla extract, and salt over low heat. Stir until well combined. Pour mixture into the prepared baking dish. Freezing it for 30 minutes will help it become firm. Slice and serve.

7.Cinnamon Roll Baked Oatmeal

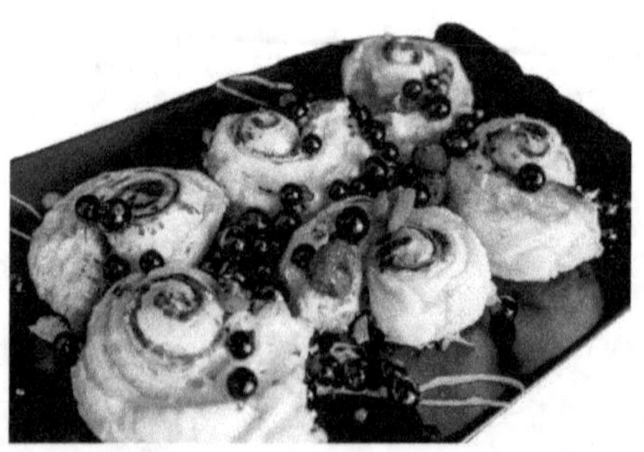

Ingredients: oats, almond milk, eggs, honey, cinnamon, baking powder, salt, cream cheese, maple syrup

Directions: Preheat oven to 375°F. Line a baking dish 8x8 inch with parchment paper. In a large bowl, mix together oats, almond milk, eggs, honey, cinnamon, baking powder, and salt until well combined. Pour mixture into the prepared baking dish. Mix the cream cheese and maple syrup in another bowl. Spoon mixture over the oats mixture. Bake for 25-30 minutes until set. Serve warm.

CHAPTER EIGHT

Conclusion

Eating well with Type 1 Diabetes can seem like a challenging task, but with the right strategies and resources, it can be manageable and even enjoyable. This cookbook has provided a comprehensive introduction to meal planning and management for those with Type 1 Diabetes, including information on understanding carbohydrates and blood sugar management, as well as delicious and easy-to-follow recipes for every meal and snack.

Recap of Meal Planning and Management Strategies:

- Understanding how carbohydrates affect blood sugar levels
- Incorporating balanced meals and snacks into your daily routine
- Making use of carb counting and other strategies to manage blood sugar levels
- Preparing meals and snacks in advance to make eating healthy more convenient
- Finding healthy options for treats and desserts

Final Thoughts on Eating for Type 1 Diabetes:
Eating well with Type 1 Diabetes requires dedication, effort, and a willingness to make changes. However, the benefits are well worth it. A healthy and balanced diet can help improve blood sugar control, boost energy levels, and promote overall health and well-being. With the information and recipes in this cookbook, you can make meal planning and management a manageable and enjoyable part of your life.

Encouragement for a Healthy Lifestyle:
Managing Type 1 Diabetes is a lifelong journey that requires commitment and effort. However, with the right tools and support, it is possible to live a happy, healthy, and fulfilling life. Take the time to learn about your condition, work closely with your healthcare provider, and make changes as necessary to improve your health.

A Final Word from the Author

Thank you for choosing this cookbook as a resource for managing Type 1 Diabetes. I hope that you have found the information and recipes helpful and that they have provided you with the tools and inspiration you need to make healthy eating a part of your daily routine. Remember, taking care of your health is a lifelong journey, and I encourage you to continue learning, growing, and making changes as necessary.